YOUR KNOWLEDGE HAS VALUE

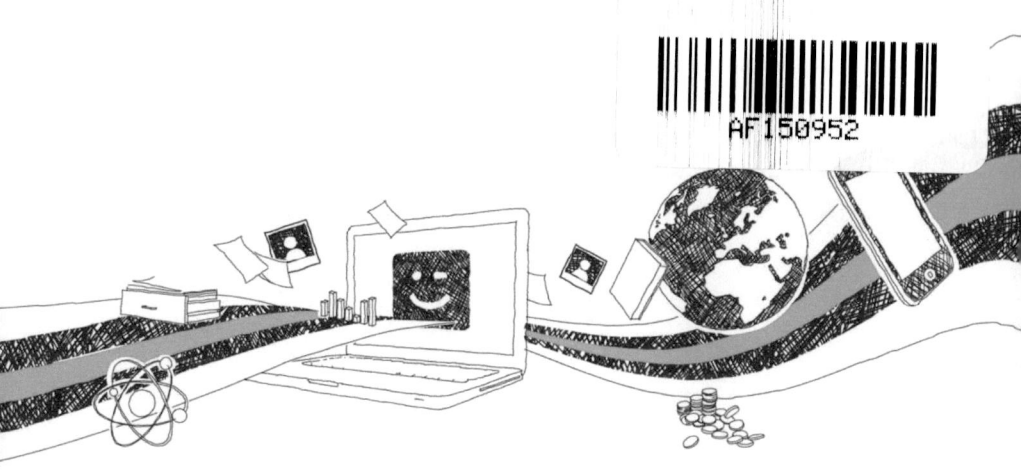
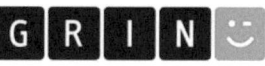

Yaw Boateng

Prevalence of Hepatitis B among the Workers of Soko-ban Wood Village in Kumasi, Ghana

GRIN Publishing

Bibliographic information published by the German National Library:

The German National Library lists this publication in the National Bibliography; detailed bibliographic data are available on the Internet at http://dnb.dnb.de .

Imprint:

Copyright © 2014 GRIN Verlag GmbH
Print and binding: Books on Demand GmbH, Norderstedt Germany
ISBN: 978-3-656-84196-8

GRIN - Your knowledge has value

Since its foundation in 1998, GRIN has specialized in publishing academic texts by students, college teachers and other academics as e-book and printed book. The website www.grin.com is an ideal platform for presenting term papers, final papers, scientific essays, dissertations and specialist books.

Visit us on the internet:

http://www.grin.com/

http://www.facebook.com/grincom

http://www.twitter.com/grin_com

PREVALENCE OF HEPATITIS B AMONG THE WORKERS OF SOKOBAN WOOD VILLAGE IN KUMASI GHANA

Boateng Yaw, Addai Theophilus and Okyere Collins. Medicare College of Applied Sciences, Department of medical laboratory technology, Pankrono, Kumasi, Ghana.

Corresponding author: Boateng Yaw (yaw.boateng@disciples.com)

ABSTRACT

Hepatitis B is still a threat to many lives in Ghana but data from non-clinical environments can be hardly found especially in Ghana. There was therefore the need for such a data to be made available and this study contributed to solving that problem. Management of the company informed the workers and those who were interested decided to join. There was a samples size of 75 workers obtained after the study. A questionnaire was administered to enable us get information on their age, marital status, history of hepatitis in family, history of blood transfusion, condom usage and history of intravenous drug use. The test was done using a HBsAg test strip from ABON i.e trademark name. The results indicated that there was a general prevalence rate of 21%. Also among those who use condoms, it was 15%. Based on marital statuses 31% of those who were positive were married, 69% were single while none was divorced. The general prevalence rate of 21% is alarming when compared to the national prevalence rate of 10 -15% and preventive measures should be put in place to curb the situation. Those who used condoms were also at risk whiles the single was the most at risk in terms of their marital statuses. Management of the company and other organisations should take it up to vaccinate the workers who were negative and also in treating those who were positive.

1.0   INTRODUCTION

1.1   Background

Hepatitis means inflammation of the liver and it is caused by the hepatitis virus. One type of hepatitis which affects the liver is hepatitis B. Hepatitis B virus (HBV) is a major cause of chronic liver disease and it affects more than 3500 million people worldwide (Wright, 2006). HBV-related chronic liver disease results in more than one million annual deaths (WHO, 2007). The infection can be transmitted through various route, that is, sexual, oral, contact with infected blood or body fluid and vertical transmission (Simonsen et al., 1999).

1.2   Problem statement

Hepatitis B virus (HBV) infection is a serious global health problem affecting 2 billion people world-wide and 350 million people suffer from chronic HBV infection (Dhawan et al., 2008). Even with three effective vaccines available, hepatitis B remains a stubborn, unrelenting health problem, especially in Africa and other developing areas. The disease and its complications cause an estimated one million deaths globally each year (Seo et al., 2008). Data from non-clinical environments can be hardly found in Ghana and with this, there is therefore the need for such a data to be made available.

1.3   Justification

Hepatitis B seems to be one of the important viruses of concern which calls for attention worldwide. The virus affects all age groups provided they come in contact with the virus when the appropriate conditions that help in the virus transmission are present. Workers of Sokoban wood village are made up of the youth who are the productive part of the economy and belong to the age group that is mostly affected by the HBV. The study on hepatitis B in Ghana is mostly limited to clinical certain and mostly done on blood donors. There is also the need for studies in various working areas or groups so as to

2

ascertain the prevalence rate among them so that appropriate steps are taking to help both those who are not infected and those who are affected. In doing that, data could also be provided for non-clinical environments.

1.4   Aims and objectives

The main aim of the study is to determine the prevalence of hepatitis B among the workers of Sokoban wood village.

1.4.1   Specific objectives

- To determine the general prevalence rate of hepatitis B among the wood workers
- To determine the effect of use of condoms on the prevalence rate of hepatitis B among the wood workers.
- To determine the prevalence of hepatitis B among wood workers who have history of blood transfusion.

2.0   MATERIALS AND METHODS

2.1   Study site

Sokoban Wood Village Enclave (SWVE) is an industrial cluster which holds an enviable place in sub-Saharan African cluster of industrial estates and its potential is well recognized as an important sector of national development. The Sokoban Wood Village Enclave is Ghana's largest wood products manufacturing district. It is located on the outskirts of Kumasi, the capital city of the Ashanti Region. SWVE was created as a replacement for the long-established informal sector wood markets in the nearby settlements of Anloga. Wood working operations were relocated as part of a Kumasi Roads and Urban Development Project by the Government of Ghana and Agence Française de Dévelopment (ADF). The Kumasi Metropolitan Assembly (KMA) manage the industrial park which includes a 1 km access road, electricity and water supplies, 62 large manufacturing and storage sheds, an administrative block and support services such as canteens, toilets, retail outlets and parking. SWVE created a new base for approximately 5,000 wood workers who had operated for over 50 years from temporary structures in a largely unregulated environment. Re-location to the new multi-purpose built settlement was presented as an opportunity to increase productivity, enhance working conditions and to reduce environmental impacts (ADF, 2010; KMA, 2009).

The majority of the workers acquire their skills through traditional apprenticeships that involve a contractual arrangement between the apprentice or the parent/guardian and the master craftsman (Adams, 2008).

2.2 Questionnaire administration

A questionnaire was administered before the tests were done. It was to enable us get information on their age, marital status, history of hepatitis in family, history of blood transfusion, condom usage and history of intravenous drug use so they were asked as such. It was one of the prerequisites needed before the test was done.

2.3 Sample collection and testing

As part of the requirements made by the management of Sokoban wood village for their workers to voluntarily know their hepatitis B status, those who were ready for them to be tested were included in the study. At the end 75 workers were involved so capillary blood was taken from the fingertip after the thumb was cleaned with alcohol. Micropipette was then used to collect 20 µl of blood which was then dropped unto the sample collection part of the test strip. Two drops of the buffer which comes with the test strip was the dropped unto the blood on the strip. The test strip which was used for the qualitative detection of HBsAg in the whole blood was manufactured by ABON which is the trademark name. It was then placed on a non-absorbent surface and result was read

4

in 15 min. The results were then interpreted as follows:

Two distinct red lines appear----POSITIVE

One red line appears in the control area----------NEAGATIVE

Control line fails to appear--------INVALID

2.4 Principles behind test strip performance

The test strip is a qualitative lateral flow immunoassay for the detection of HBsAg in serum or plasma. The membrane is pre-coated with anti-HBsAg antibodies on the test line region of the strip. During the testing, the serum or plasma specimen reacts with the particle coated with anti-HBsAg antibody. The mixture migrates upward on the membrane chromatographically by capillary action to react with anti-HBsAg on the membrane and generate a coloured. The presence of this coloured line in the test region indicates a positive result, while its absence indicate a negative result. To serve as a procedural control, a coloured line will always appear in the control line region indicating that proper volume of specimen has been added and membrane wicking has occurred.

2.5 Limitations of test strip performance

The HBsAg one step Hepatitis B Surface Antigen only indicate the presence of HBsAg in the specimen and should not be used as the sole criteria for the diagnosis of Hepatitis B virus infection. Also all diagnostic tests results must be considered with other clinical information. Lastly, the One Step Hepatitis B Surface Antigen Test Strip cannot detect less than I ng/ml of HBsAg in specimens.

3.0 RESULTS AND DISCUSSIONS

3.1 Questionnaire

From the questionnaire it was realised that 26.7% of the wood workers had history of hepatitis in family with the majority not having such a history. Since hepatitis B can be transmitted from parents to their offspring during birth, there was therefore the need for such information to be asked so that it will help in giving a clue of the disease in a workers family especially those who were positive.

On the history of blood transfusion, 85.7% of the workers said no and so this means the rest (13.3%) had been transfused with blood before. Screening of blood is one of the major means of preventing transmission of the infection to healthy individuals so there is the need for proper screening of blood to be done. Also screening of blood for hepatitis B in Ghana started in the early 90's so those who were transfused with blood before the said date risk been infected so there was therefore the need for this information to be obtained from the wood workers.

It was realised that majority of the respondents (57.3%) were single, 40% were married whiles 2.7% had divorced. Since the disease can be transmitted from one couple to the other, there was therefore the need for these statuses to be known so that if they are positive their partners and children could also be tested and advised.

Condom use is one of the means of preventing hepatitis B from one person to the other through sex and from the study it was realised that 61.3% of the wood workers who took part in the study use condoms whiles 37.7% do not use them but as to why they don't use them should be another study. Though use of condoms can prevent hepatitis B from been transmitted from one partner to the other, it is not the only means preventing the disease from been transmitted from one person to the other but other means exists.

6

Though intravenous drug use is not very common in our part of the country, it is one of the ways of contracting hepatitis B especially if one of those sharing the needle is infected. It was realised from the study that only 8% had such history while 92% which was the majority had no such history.

3.2 General prevalence of hepatitis B among the wood workers

At the end of the study a prevalence rate of 21% was obtained as represented in Fig 2. This rate is high when compared to the national prevalence rate of between 10 – 15%. That makes it serious and it calls for attention from all stakeholders who are interested in the prevention of hepatitis B. This is also the highly productive ones due to their age and with time it will affect the output of their work. A study conducted by Muhammad *et al.* (2012) on hepatitis B prevalence among factory workers of Gujranwala district of Punjab province (Pakistan) came out with a prevalence rate

of 3.8% and this tells us that the issue of Sokoban wood village workers is highly alarming and calls for immediate attention.

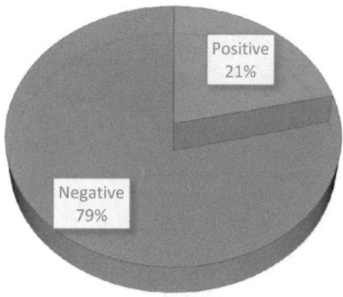

Fig. 2 Prevalence of hepatitis B among the workers of Sokoban wood village

3.3 Prevalence of hepatitis B among condom users

Condom use which is one of the preventive ways of hepatitis B had a prevalence of 15% among its users. This suggests that though they use these condoms to prevent them from getting hepatitis B, there are other ways they can get the disease and they could have probably gotten it from the other modes of infection. Also 85% of the wood workers who used the condoms had negative and this could probably due to its use otherwise the prevalence rate would have been higher than what has been obtained.

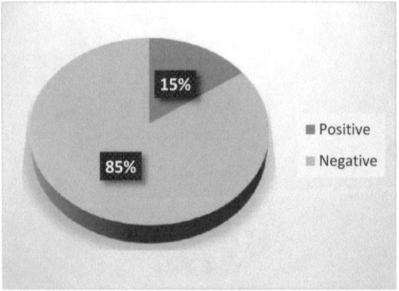

Fig. 3 Prevalence rate among wood workers who use condoms

3.4   Prevalence of hepatitis B based on marital statuses

Among the 40% who were married, there was a prevalence rate of 16.7%. Also the majority who were singles had 25.6% of them been positive. Lastly, 2.7% were divorced and there was no positive case among the divorced.

This suggests that prevalence rate among the singles was overwhelming and there is a need for it to be of concern. Since, they

are not married they should be probably be advised to be protective of themselves against the disease. The married also has an issue of concern since they might probably infect their wives and children if the virus is at its infective stage.

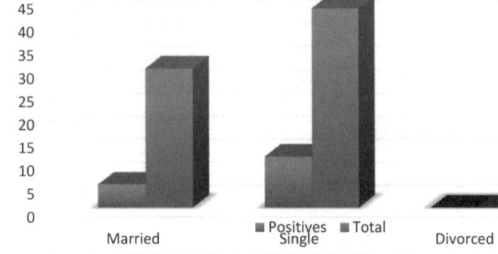

Based on the marital statuses for those who were positive, 31% were married while 69% were singles with none for them divorced as represented in Fig. 5.

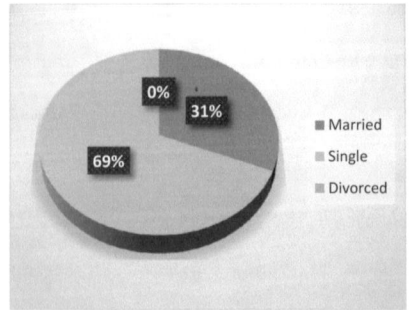

Fig. 5 Prevalence based on marital status of the wood workers

Fig. 6 Prevalence among those with history of hepatitis in family

3.5 Prevalence of hepatitis B among those with history of hepatitis in family

Those who had histories of hepatitis B in family which might lead to them getting infected especially through birth, recorded a prevalence rate of 50% as has been resented in Fig. 6. This tells us that there are a lot of people who might have gotten the virus from family and in this case from their mothers during birth. One other issue of concern too is that these people who get when they are below 5 years become chronic according to WHO. This therefore calls for attention since hepatitis B infection among family members can be very serious.

3.6 Prevalence of hepatitis B among those with history of blood transfusion

Blood transfusion can lead to transmission of the virus to a healthy individual and among those who had received blood transfusions before, 20% were positive for the hepatitis B virus. Though there are not enough evidence to suggest that the virus was obtained through the blood transfusion, it could have probably been the case especially with those who received these transfusions before early 1990s since before that time they were not screened for the virus. It could probably also happen that the test was done but not properly with confirmatory test like ELISA or PCR since most of our labs do not do it.

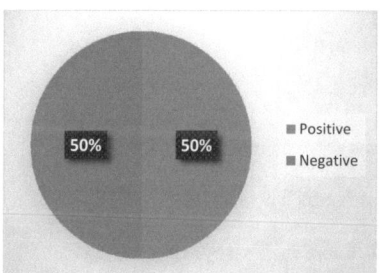

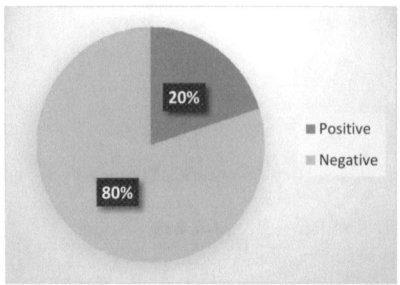

Fig. 7 Prevalence among workers with history of blood transfusion

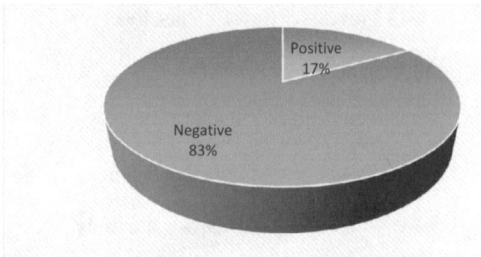

Fig. 7 Prevalence among those workers with intravenous drug use

3.7 Prevalence of hepatitis B among those with history of intravenous drug use

Drug use especially the narcotics intravenously among people who do not ensure safe practice can lead to the spread of the virus from one person the other. It was revealed that among the 8% of the total population who were victims to that, 17% were positive. This suggests that they could have probably gotten the virus from the use of the intravenous drugs.

4.0 CONCLUSION AND RECOMMENDATIONS

4.1 Conclusion

The effect of hepatitis B globally cannot be neglected due to the fact that it has been claiming many lives of all ages. Therefore this study was to determine the prevalence rate of the disease among wood workers of Sokoban wood village. There were 75 workers involved in the study as they did it voluntarily as was requested by the management of the area.

There was a prevalence rate of 21% among the workers which is more than the national prevalence rate of 10 -15% from different studies. The prevalence rate among condom users was 15%, prevalence among the married was 16.7%, singles was 25%, the divorced was none, those with history of hepatitis in family was 50%, those with history of blood transfusion was 20% and those with intravenous drug use was 16.7%.

These prevalence rates call for attention and all stakeholders should put in efforts to help solve the problem. Confirmatory tests such as PCR and ELISA should be done. Further tests such as liver function, hepatitis B profile and viral load should be done for those positive workers whiles those negative individuals should be vaccinated.

4.2   Recommendation

The study has been effective in revealing the prevalence rate of hepatitis B among the wood workers of Sokoban wood village and based on the experience and results obtained during the study these recommendations have been made.

There the need for the management of the Sokoban wood village to sponsor or make it compulsory for all who were negative during the testing to be vaccinated for there is the saying that prevention is better cure. Also those who were negative should be assisted in checking their liver function, hepatitis B profile and viral load so as to establish the extent and stage of the disease in the positive individuals.

It also recommended that further confirmatory tests such as PCR and ELISA should be done as confirmatory tests. Due to financial constraints, this study could not go further to do that but future studies should consider such confirmatory tests.

Due to the high prevalence rate obtained during this study, it is suggested that other working areas should be involved in such studies so that the prevalence rate at various working areas will be obtained locally and that will help in the preventative steps that can be put in place.

REFERENCES

KMA, (2009). Sokoban Wood Village - handing over report. Kumasi: Kumasi Metropolitan Assembly.

Muhammad I., Muhammad I., Usman R. and Shazia Y. (2012). Prevalence of Hepatitis B virus infection among population of factory workers in Gujranwala (Punjab) Pakistan

Simonsen L, Kane A, Lloyd J, Zaffran M, Kane M. (1999). Unsafe injections in the developing world and transmission of blood-borne pathogens: a review. Bull. World Health Organ., 77(10): 789-800.

Seo H.S., Park J.S., Han K.Y., Bae K.D., Ahn S.J., Kang H.A. and Lee J. (2008). Analysis and characterization of hepatitis B vaccine particles synthesized from *Hansenula polymorpha*. Vaccine, 26(33), 4138-4144.

World Health Organization (2007). Department of Communicable Disease Surveillance and Response, author; Hepatitis B.

Wright T.L. (2006). Introduction to chronic hepatitis B infection. Am. J. Gastroenterol., 101(Suppl 1): S1-6.

.